Content

Introduction

The DASH diet, which stands for dietary approaches to stop hypertension, is promoted by the National Heart, Lung and Blood Institute to do exactly that: stop (or prevent) hypertension, aka high blood pressure. It emphasizes the foods you've always been told to eat (fruits, veggies, whole grains, lean protein and low-fat dairy), which are high in blood pressure-deflating nutrients like potassium, calcium, protein and fiber.

This research also discourages foods that are high in saturated fat, such as fatty meats, full-fat dairy foods and tropical oils, as well as sugar-sweetened beverages and sweets. Consuming entire grain was also revealed to lover blood pressure and consuming lean meat can replace into healthy protein consumption. This can be advantage over popular protein sources such as red meat and pork.

This book will help you manage and regulate Completely your high blood pressure.

What is the DASH diet?

The DASH diet, which stands for dietary approaches to stop hypertension, is promoted by the National Heart, Lung and Blood Institute to do exactly that: stop (or prevent) hypertension, aka high blood pressure. It emphasizes the foods you've always been told to eat (fruits, veggies, whole grains, lean protein and low-fat dairy), which are high in blood pressure-deflating nutrients like potassium, calcium, protein and fiber.

DASH also discourages foods that are high in saturated fat, such as fatty meats, full-fat dairy foods and tropical oils, as well as sugar-sweetened beverages and sweets.

The DASH eating plan

DASH Food Groups:

Vegetables

Fruit

Grains (mainly whole grains)

Low Fat or No-Fat Dairy Foods

Lean meats, poultry and fish

Nuts, seeds and dry beans

Fats and Oils

DASH Daily Servings (except as noted) and examples:

Vegetables: 4-5 servings

250 mL (1 cup) raw leafy vegetables

125 mL (½ cup) cooked vegetables

Fruit: 4-5 servings

1 medium piece of fruit

63 mL (¼ cup) dried fruit

125 mL (½ cup) fresh, frozen or canned fruit

Grains (mainly whole grains): 7-8 servings

1 slice bread

250 mL (1 cup) ready to eat cereal

125 mL (½ cup) cooked rice, pasta or cereal

Low Fat or No-Fat Dairy Foods: 2-3 servings

250 mL (1 cup) milk

250 mL (1 cup) yogurt

50 g (1½ oz) cheese

Lean meats, poultry and fish: 2 servings or less

3 ounces cooked lean meats, skinless poultry, or fish

Nuts, seeds and dry beans: 4-5 servings per week

1/3 cup (1.5 oz.) nuts

30 mL (2 tbsp) peanut butter

2 tbsp (1/2 oz.) seeds

1/2 cup cooked dry beans or peas

Fats and oils: 2-3 servings

5 mL (1 tsp) soft margarine

15mL (1 tbsp) low-fat mayonnaise

30 mL (2 tbsp) light salad dressing

5 mL (1 tsp) vegetable oil

What about medication?

Many people require medication to control their blood pressure. Lifestyle modification, which includes healthy eating and regular physical activity, may be the only treatment needed in those with mild high blood pressure. In those that require medication to control their blood pressure, following a healthy lifestyle may reduce the need for, or the amount of, medication required.

What next?

A full healthy lifestyle, including healthy eating, is part of the Canadian recommendations for the management of high blood pressure. Heart and Stroke is involved in developing blood pressure guidelines, which are updated every year. To control your blood pressure and reduce the risk of heart disease, the guidelines recommend that you:

Be active 30 to 60 minutes most days of the week.

Choose the following more often: vegetables, fruit, low-fat dairy or dairy alternatives, whole grains and protein from a variety of foods, such as beans, lentils, nuts and seeds, lean meats, poultry and fish. Limit fast foods, processed foods because they usually have more sodium and saturated fat.

If you are overweight, losing about 10 lb (5 kg) will lower your blood pressure. Reducing your weight to within a healthy range for your age and gender will lower your blood pressure even more.

Eat less salt by:

limiting your use of salt in cooking and at the table

avoiding highly processed foods

choosing fresh or plain frozen vegetables and fruit

avoiding canned or prepared foods that are high in salt

reading the Nutrition Facts table on food packages for sodium content using other seasonings such as herbs, spices, lemon juice and garlic during food preparation

If you drink alcohol, limit yourself to no more than 2 drinks a day, to a weekly maximum of 10 for women and 3 drinks a day to a weekly maximum of 15 for men. (Do not drink when you are driving a vehicle, taking medications or other drugs that interact with alcohol, pregnant or are planning to be pregnant, making important decisions, doing any kind of dangerous physical activity, living with alcohol dependence or mental or physical health problems, or responsible for the safety of others. If you are concerned about how drinking may affect your health, talk to your doctor).

Be smoke-free. It is important to stop smoking if you have high blood pressure. Smoking increases the risk of developing heart problems and other diseases. Your home and workplace should also be smoke-free.

Take your medication as prescribed.

Monitor your blood pressure regularly.

Avoid drinking sugar sweetened beverages. Choose safe drinking water, low fat milk or tea instead.

Changing your diet means a life-long commitment to healthier lifestyle choices. People who make small changes in their diet over a longer period of time, rather than a dramatic change all at once, are more likely to stay committed to a healthier diet.

If you are considering starting on the DASH diet, discuss it with your healthcare provider first.

How much salt?

We recommend Canadians consume no more than 2,300 mg of sodium (about 1 teaspoon/5 mL of table salt) a day. The amount of salt you eat isn't just what you shake onto your food – it is already added in large quantities to prepared foods, canned products, snack foods and restaurant meals.

2 ways to get started on the DASH diet

Change gradually:

If you now eat one or two vegetables a day, add another serving at lunch and dinner.

If you don't eat fruit now or have only juice at breakfast, add a serving of fruit to your meals or switch out your juice for the whole fruit.

Limit meat and alternatives to about 6 oz (170 g) over two meals (two servings). Each serving is about the size of a deck of cards or the palm of your hand.

Choose plant-based proteins more often.

Choose fruit, vegetables, whole grains or protein foods for desserts and snacks.

Choose a variety of foods

In the DASH-Sodium study, participants were given one of three sodium plans: the DASH diet with 3,300 mg of sodium per day (a normal amount for many North Americans); 2,300 mg of sodium (a moderately restricted amount); or 1,500 mg of sodium (a more restricted amount, about 2/3 of a teaspoon of salt). Blood pressure was lower for everyone on the DASH diet. However, the less salt people consumed, the greater the decrease in blood pressure. People who already had high blood pressure had the largest decrease in blood pressure.

Why is a healthy blood pressure important?

High blood pressure causes the heart to work harder to pump nutrient- and oxygen-rich blood to the body. The arteries that deliver the blood become scarred and less elastic. Although these changes happen to everyone as they age, they happen more quickly in people with high blood pressure. As the arteries stiffen, the heart has to work even harder, causing the heart muscle to become thicker, weaker and less able to pump blood. When high blood pressure damages arteries, they are not able to deliver enough blood to organs for their proper functioning. As a result, organs may become damaged, too. For example, this type of damage can affect the heart, causing a heart attack, the brain, causing a stroke, and the kidneys, leading to kidney failure.

How is DASH different from Canadian recommendations?

The DASH diet isn't unique – it is very similar to Canada's Food Guide.

Both Canada's Food Guide and the DASH diet focus on vegetables, fruit, whole grains and protein choices such as nuts, seeds, beans, lean meats, poultry, fish and low- fat dairy foods. The DASH diet is also low in saturated fat, sugar and salt.

Canada's Food Guide has moved away from specific serving sizes to the plate method. At every meal fill half your plate with vegetables and fruit, a quarter of your plate with whole-grain foods, and a quarter of your plate with protein foods. The DASH diet specifies the number of servings and serving sizes for each food group.

High blood pressure affects more than a billion people worldwide — and that number is rising.

In fact, the number of people with high blood pressure has doubled in the last 40 years — a serious health concern, as high blood pressure is linked to a higher risk of conditions such as heart disease, kidney failure and stroke (1Trusted Source, 2Trusted Source).

As diet is thought to play a major role in the development of high blood pressure, scientists and policymakers have engineered specific dietary strategies to help reduce it (3Trusted Source, 4Trusted Source).

This article examines the DASH diet, which was designed to combat high blood pressure and reduce people's risk of heart disease.

What Is the DASH Diet?

Dietary Approaches to Stop Hypertension, or DASH, is a diet recommended for people who want to prevent or treat hypertension — also known as high blood pressure — and reduce their risk of heart disease.

The DASH diet focuses on fruits, vegetables, whole grains and lean meats.

The diet was created after researchers noticed that high blood pressure was much less common in people who followed a plant-based diet, such as vegans and vegetarians (5Trusted Source, 6Trusted Source).

That's why the DASH diet emphasizes fruits and vegetables while containing some lean protein sources like chicken, fish and beans. The diet is low in red meat, salt, added sugars and fat.

Scientists believe that one of the main reasons people with high blood pressure can benefit from this diet is because it reduces salt intake.

The regular DASH diet program encourages no more than 1 teaspoon (2,300 mg) of sodium per day, which is in line with most national guidelines.

The lower-salt version recommends no more than 3/4 teaspoon (1,500 mg) of sodium per day.

SUMMARY

The DASH diet was designed to reduce high blood pressure. While rich in fruits, vegetables and lean proteins, it restricts red meat, salt, added sugars and fat.

Potential Benefits

Beyond reducing blood pressure, the DASH diet offers a number of potential benefits, including weight loss and reduced cancer risk.

However, you shouldn't expect DASH to help you shed weight on its own — as it was designed fundamentally to lower blood pressure. Weight loss may simply be an added perk.

The diet impacts your body in several ways.

Lowers Blood Pressure

Blood pressure is a measure of the force put on your blood vessels and organs as your blood passes through them. It's counted in two numbers:

Systolic pressure: The pressure in your blood vessels when your heart beats.

Diastolic pressure: The pressure in your blood vessels between heartbeats, when your heart is at rest.

Normal blood pressure for adults is a systolic pressure below 120 mmHg and a diastolic pressure below 80 mmHg. This is normally written with the systolic blood pressure above the diastolic pressure, like this: 120/80.

People with a blood pressure reading of 140/90 are considered to have high blood pressure.

Interestingly, the DASH diet demonstrably lowers blood pressure in both healthy people and those with high blood pressure.

In studies, people on the DASH diet still experienced lower blood pressure even if they didn't lose weight or restrict salt intake (7Trusted Source, 8Trusted Source).

However, when sodium intake was restricted, the DASH diet lowered blood pressure even further. In fact, the greatest reductions in blood pressure were seen in people with the lowest salt consumption (9Trusted Source).

These low-salt DASH diet results were most impressive in people who already had high blood pressure, reducing systolic blood pressure by an average of 12 mmHg and diastolic blood pressure by 5 mmHg (5Trusted Source).

In people with normal blood pressure, it reduced systolic blood pressure by 4 mmHg and diastolic by 2 mmHg (5Trusted Source).

This is in line with other studies which reveal that restricting salt intake can reduce blood pressure — especially in those who have high blood pressure (10Trusted Source).

Keep in mind that a decrease in blood pressure does not always translate to a decreased risk of heart disease (11Trusted Source).

May Aid Weight Loss

You will likely experience lower blood pressure on the DASH diet whether or not you lose weight.

However, if you already have high blood pressure, chances are you have been advised to lose weight.

This is because the more you weigh, the higher your blood pressure is likely to be (12Trusted Source, 13Trusted Source, 14Trusted Source).

Additionally, losing weight has been shown to lower blood pressure (15Trusted Source, 16Trusted Source).

Some studies suggest that people can lose weight on the DASH diet (17Trusted Source, 18Trusted Source, 19Trusted Source).

However, those who have lost weight on the DASH diet have been in a controlled calorie deficit — meaning they were told to eat fewer calories than they were expending.

Given that the DASH diet cuts out a lot of high-fat, sugary foods, people may find that they automatically reduce their calorie intake and lose weight. Other people may have to consciously restrict their intake (20Trusted Source).

Either way, if you want to lose weight on the DASH diet, you'll still need to go on a calorie-reduced diet.

Other Potential Health Benefits

DASH may also affect other areas of health. The diet:

Decreases cancer risk: A recent review indicated that people following the DASH diet had a lower risk of some cancers, including colorectal and breast cancer.

Lowers metabolic syndrome risk: Some studies note that the DASH diet reduces your risk of metabolic syndrome by up to 81%.

Lowers diabetes risk: The diet has been linked to a lower risk of type 2 diabetes. Some studies demonstrate that it can improve insulin resistance as well.

Decreases heart disease risk: In one recent review in women, following a DASH-like diet was associated with a 20% lower risk of heart disease and a 29% lower risk of stroke (26Trusted Source).

Many of these protective effects are attributed to the diet's high fruit and vegetable content. In general, eating more fruits and vegetables can help reduce risk of disease.

SUMMARY

DASH lowers blood pressure — particularly if you have elevated levels — and may aid weight loss. It could reduce your risk of diabetes, heart disease, metabolic syndrome and some cancers.

Does It Work for Everyone?

While studies on the DASH diet determined that the greatest reductions in blood pressure occurred in those with the lowest salt intake, the benefits of salt restriction on health and lifespan are not clear-cut.

For people with high blood pressure, reducing salt intake significantly affects blood pressure. However, in people with normal blood pressure, the effects of reducing salt intake are much smaller (6Trusted Source, 10Trusted Source).

The theory that some people are salt sensitive — meaning that salt exerts a greater influence on their blood pressure — could partly explain this.

SUMMARY

If your salt intake is high, lowering it can offer major health benefits. Comprehensive salt restriction, as advised on the DASH diet, may only be beneficial for people who are salt sensitive or have high blood pressure.

Restricting Salt Too Much Is Not Good for You

Eating too little salt has been linked to health problems, such as an increased risk of heart disease, insulin resistance and fluid retention.

The low-salt version of the DASH diet recommends that people eat no more than 3/4 teaspoon (1,500 mg) of sodium per day.

However, it's unclear whether there are any benefits to reducing salt intake this low — even in people with high blood pressure.

In fact, a recent review found no link between salt intake and risk of death from heart disease, despite the fact that lowering salt intake caused a modest reduction in blood pressure.

However, because most people eat too much salt, lowering your salt intake from very high amounts of 2–2.5 teaspoons (10–12 grams) a day to 1–1.25 teaspoons (5–6 grams) a day may be beneficial.

This target can be achieved easily by reducing the amount of highly processed food in your diet and eating mostly whole foods.

SUMMARY

Although reducing salt intake from processed foods is beneficial for most people, eating too little salt may also be harmful.

What to Eat on the Diet

The DASH diet doesn't list specific foods to eat.

Instead, it recommends specific servings of different food groups.

The number of servings you can eat depends on how many calories you consume. Below is an example of food portions based on a 2,000-calorie diet.

Whole Grains: 6–8 Servings per Day

Examples of whole grains include whole-wheat or whole-grain breads, whole-grain breakfast cereals, brown rice, bulgur, quinoa and oatmeal.

Examples of a serving include:

1 slice of whole-grain bread

1 ounce (28 grams) of dry, whole-grain cereal

1/2 cup (95 grams) of cooked rice, pasta or cereal

Vegetables: 4–5 Servings per Day

All vegetables are allowed on the DASH diet.

Examples of a serving include:

1 cup (about 30 grams) of raw, leafy green vegetables like spinach or kale

1/2 cup (about 45 grams) of sliced vegetables — raw or cooked — like broccoli, carrots, squash or tomatoes

Fruits: 4–5 Servings per Day

If you're following the DASH approach, you'll be eating a lot of fruit. Examples of fruits you can eat include apples, pears, peaches, berries and tropical fruits like pineapple and mango.

Examples of a serving include:

1 medium apple

1/4 cup (50 grams) of dried apricots

1/2 cup (30 grams) of fresh, frozen or canned peaches

Dairy Products: 2–3 Servings per Day

Dairy products on the DASH diet should be low in fat.

Examples include skim milk and low-fat cheese and yogurt.

Examples of a serving include:

1 cup (240 ml) of low-fat milk

1 cup (285 grams) of low-fat yogurt

1.5 ounces (45 grams) of low-fat cheese

Lean Chicken, Meat and Fish: 6 or Fewer Servings per Day

Choose lean cuts of meat and try to eat a serving of red meat

only occasionally — no more than once or twice a week.

Examples of a serving include:

1 ounce (28 grams) of cooked meat, chicken or fish

1 egg

Nuts, Seeds and Legumes: 4–5 Servings per Week

These include almonds, peanuts, hazelnuts, walnuts, sunflower seeds, flaxseeds, kidney beans, lentils and split peas.

Examples of a serving include:

1/3 cup (50 grams) of nuts

2 tablespoons (40 grams) of nut butter

2 tablespoons (16 grams) of seeds

1/2 cup (40 grams) of cooked legumes

Fats and Oils: 2–3 Servings per Day

The DASH diet recommends vegetable oils over other oils. These include margarines and oils like canola, corn, olive or safflower. It also recommends low-fat mayonnaise and light salad dressing.

Examples of a serving include:

1 teaspoon (4.5 grams) of soft margarine

1 teaspoon (5 ml) of vegetable oil

1 tablespoon (15 grams) of mayonnaise

2 tablespoons (30 ml) of salad dressing

Candy and Added Sugars: 5 or Fewer Servings per Week

Added sugars are kept to a minimum on the DASH diet, so limit your intake of candy, soda and table sugar. The DASH diet also restricts unrefined sugars and alternative sugar sources, like agave nectar.

Examples of a serving include:

1 tablespoon (12.5 grams) of sugar

1 tablespoon (20 grams) of jelly or jam

1 cup (240 ml) of lemonade

SUMMARY

The DASH diet does not list specific foods to eat. Instead, it's a dietary pattern focused on servings of food groups.

Sample Menu for One Week

Here's an example of a one-week meal plan — based on 2,000 calories per day — for the regular DASH diet:

Monday

Breakfast: 1 cup (90 grams) of oatmeal with 1 cup (240 ml) of skim milk, 1/2 cup (75 grams) of blueberries and 1/2 cup (120 ml) of fresh orange juice.

Snack: 1 medium apple and 1 cup (285 grams) of low-fat yogurt.

Lunch: Tuna and mayonnaise sandwich made with 2 slices of whole-grain bread, 1 tablespoon (15 grams) of mayonnaise, 1.5 cups (113 grams) of green salad and 3 ounces (80 grams) of canned tuna.

Snack: 1 medium banana.

Dinner: 3 ounces (85 grams) of lean chicken breast cooked in 1 teaspoon (5 ml) of vegetable oil with 1/2 cup (75 grams) each of broccoli and carrots. Served with 1 cup (190 grams) of brown rice.

Tuesday

Breakfast: 2 slices of whole-wheat toast with 1 teaspoon (4.5 grams) of margarine, 1 tablespoon (20 grams) of jelly or jam, 1/2 cup (120 ml) of fresh orange juice and 1 medium apple.

Snack: 1 medium banana.

Lunch: 3 ounces (85 grams) of lean chicken breast with 2 cups (150 grams) of green salad, 1.5 ounces (45 grams) of low-fat cheese and 1 cup (190 grams) of brown rice.

Snack: 1/2 cup (30 grams) of canned peaches and 1 cup (285 grams) of low-fat yogurt.

Dinner: 3 ounces (85 grams) of salmon cooked in 1 teaspoon (5 ml) of vegetable oil with 1 cup (300 grams) of boiled potatoes and 1.5 cups (225 grams) of boiled vegetables.

Wednesday

Breakfast: 1 cup (90 grams) of oatmeal with 1 cup (240 ml) of skim milk and 1/2 cup (75 grams) of blueberries. 1/2 cup (120 ml) of fresh orange juice.

Snack: 1 medium orange.

Lunch: 2 slices of whole-wheat bread, 3 ounces (85 grams) of lean turkey, 1.5 ounces (45 grams) of low-fat cheese, 1/2 cup

(38 grams) of green salad and 1/2 cup (38 grams) of cherry tomatoes.

Snack: 4 whole-grain crackers with 1.5 ounces (45 grams) of cottage cheese and 1/2 cup (75 grams) of canned pineapple.

Dinner: 6 ounces (170 grams) of cod fillet, 1 cup (200 grams) of mashed potatoes, 1/2 cup (75 grams) of green peas and 1/2 cup (75 grams) of broccoli.

Thursday

Breakfast: 1 cup (90 grams) of oatmeal with 1 cup (240 ml) of skim milk and 1/2 cup (75 grams) of raspberries. 1/2 cup (120 ml) of fresh orange juice.

Snack: 1 medium banana.

Lunch: Salad made with 4.5 ounces (130 grams) of grilled tuna, 1 boiled egg, 2 cups (152 grams) of green salad, 1/2 cup (38 grams) of cherry tomatoes and 2 tablespoons (30 ml) of low-fat dressing.

Snack: 1/2 cup (30 grams) of canned pears and 1 cup (285 grams) of low-fat yogurt.

Dinner: 3 ounces (85 grams) of pork fillet with 1 cup (150 grams) of mixed vegetables and 1 cup (190 grams) of brown rice.

Friday

Breakfast: 2 boiled eggs, 2 slices of turkey bacon with 1/2 cup (38 grams) of cherry tomatoes, 1/2 cup (80 grams) of baked beans and 2 slices of whole-wheat toast, plus 1/2 cup (120 ml) of fresh orange juice.

Snack: 1 medium apple.

Lunch: 2 slices of whole-wheat toast, 1 tablespoon of low-fat mayonnaise, 1.5 ounces (45 grams) of low-fat cheese, 1/2 cup (38 grams) of salad greens and 1/2 cup (38 grams) of cherry tomatoes.

Snack: 1 cup of fruit salad.

Dinner: Spaghetti and meatballs made with 1 cup (190 grams) of spaghetti and 4 ounces (115 grams) of minced turkey. 1/2 cup (75 grams) of green peas on the side.

Saturday

Breakfast: 2 slices of whole-wheat toast with 2 tablespoons (40 grams) of peanut butter, 1 medium banana, 2 tablespoons (16 grams) of mixed seeds and 1/2 cup (120 ml) of fresh orange juice.

Snack: 1 medium apple.

Lunch: 3 ounces (85 grams) of grilled chicken, 1 cup (150 grams) of roasted vegetables and 1 cup (190 grams) couscous.

Snack: 1/2 cup (30 grams) of mixed berries and 1 cup (285 grams) of low-fat yogurt.

Dinner: 3 ounces (85 grams) of pork steak and 1 cup (150 grams) of ratatouille with 1 cup (190 grams) of brown rice,

1/2 cup (40 grams) of lentils and 1.5 ounces (45 grams) of low-fat cheese.

Dessert: Low-fat chocolate pudding.

Sunday

Breakfast: 1 cup (90 grams) of oatmeal with 1 cup (240 ml) of skim milk, 1/2 cup (75 grams) of blueberries and 1/2 cup (120 ml) of fresh orange juice.

Snack: 1 medium pear.

Lunch: Chicken salad made with 3 ounces (85 grams) of lean chicken breast, 1 tablespoon of mayonnaise, 2 cups (150 grams) of green salad, 1/2 cup (75 grams) of cherry tomatoes,

1/2 tablespoon (4 grams) of seeds and 4 whole-grain crackers.

Snack: 1 banana and 1/2 cup (70 grams) of almonds.

Dinner: 3 ounces of roast beef with 1 cup (150 grams) of boiled potatoes, 1/2 cup (75 grams) of broccoli and 1/2 cup (75 grams) of green peas.

SUMMARY

On the DASH diet, you can eat a variety of scrumptious, healthy meals that pack plenty of vegetables alongside various fruits and good protein sources.

How to Make Your Diet More DASH-Like

Because there are no set foods on the DASH diet, you can adapt your current diet to the DASH guidelines by doing the following:

Eat more vegetables and fruits.

Swap refined grains for whole grains.

Choose fat-free or low-fat dairy products.

Choose lean protein sources like fish, poultry and beans.

Cook with vegetable oils.

Limit your intake of foods high in added sugars, like soda and candy.

Limit your intake of foods high in saturated fats like fatty meats, full-fat dairy and oils like coconut and palm oil.

Outside of measured fresh fruit juice portions, this diet recommends you stick to low-calorie drinks like water, tea and coffee.

SUMMARY

It's possible to align your current diet with the DASH diet. Simply eat more fruits and vegetables, choose low-fat products as well as lean proteins and limit your intake of processed, high-fat and sugary foods.

Frequently Asked Questions

If you're thinking about trying DASH to lower your blood pressure, you might have a few questions about other aspects of your lifestyle.

The most commonly asked questions are addressed below.

Can I Drink Coffee on the DASH Diet?

The DASH diet doesn't prescribe specific guidelines for coffee. However, some people worry that caffeinated beverages like coffee may increase their blood pressure.

It's well known that caffeine can cause a short-term increase in blood pressure. For most healthy people with normal blood pressure, 3–4 regular cups of coffee per day are considered safe. Keep in mind that the slight rise in blood pressure (5–10 mm Hg) caused by caffeine means that people who already have high blood pressure probably need to be more careful with their coffee consumption.

Do I Need to Exercise on the DASH Diet?

The DASH diet is even more effective at lowering blood pressure when paired with physical activity.

Given the independent benefits of exercise on health, this is not surprising.

It's recommended to do 30 minutes of moderate activity most days, and it's important to choose something you enjoy — this way, you will be more likely to keep it up.

Examples of moderate activity include:

Brisk walking (15 minutes per mile or 9 minutes per kilometer)

Running (10 minutes per mile or 6 minutes per kilometer)

Cycling (6 minutes per mile or 4 minutes per kilometer)

Swimming laps (20 minutes)

Housework (60 minutes)

Can I Drink Alcohol on the DASH Diet?

Drinking too much alcohol can increase your blood pressure.

In fact, regularly drinking more than 3 drinks per day has been linked to an increased risk of high blood pressure and heart disease (38Trusted Source).

On the DASH diet, you should drink alcohol sparingly and not exceed official guidelines — 2 or fewer drinks per day for men and 1 or fewer for women.

SUMMARY

You can drink coffee and alcohol in moderation on the DASH diet. Combining the DASH diet with exercise may make it even more effective.

The DASH diet may be an easy and effective way to reduce blood pressure.

However, keep in mind that cutting daily salt intake to 3/4 teaspoon (1,500 mg) or less has not been linked to any hard health benefits — such as a reduced risk of heart disease — despite the fact that it can lower blood pressure.

Moreover, the DASH diet is very similar to the standard low-fat diet, which large controlled trials have not shown to reduce the risk of death by heart disease (39Trusted Source, 40Trusted Source).

Healthy individuals may have little reason to follow this diet. Nevertheless, if you have high blood pressure or think you may be sensitive to salt, DASH may be a good choice for you.

Das diet Recipes

Serves 8

High Fiber

Healthy carb

Low Sodium

Low Fat

Ingredients

1 can (15.5 ounces) artichoke hearts in water, drained

4 cups chopped raw spinach

2 cloves garlic, minced

1 teaspoon ground black pepper

1 teaspoon minced fresh thyme (or 1/3 teaspoon dried)

1 tablespoon fresh minced parsley (or 1 teaspoon dried)

1 cup prepared unsalted white beans (or half a 15.5-ounce can unsalted white beans, rinsed and drained)

2 tablespoons grated Parmesan cheese

1/2 cup low-fat sour cream

Directions

In a mixing bowl, combine the ingredients. Transfer to an oven-safe glass or ceramic dish and bake at 350 F for 30 minutes. Serve warm.

Nutritional analysis per serving

Serving size: About 1/2 cup

Total carbohydrate10 g

Dietary fiber6 g

Sodium130 mg

Saturated fat1 g

Total fat2 g

Trans fat0 g

Cholesterol6 mg

Protein5 g

Monounsaturated fatTrace

Calories78

Added sugars0 g

Total sugars1.5 g

Artichoke, spinach and white beans

Number of servings

Serves 8

Low Fat

High Fiber

Low Sodium

Healthy carb

Ingredients

2 cups artichoke hearts

1 tablespoon black pepper

4 cups chopped spinach

1 teaspoon minced dried thyme

2 cloves garlic, minced

1 tablespoon minced fresh parsley

1 cup cooked white beans

2 tablespoons grated parmesan cheese

1/2 cup reduced-fat sour cream

Directions

Heat oven to 350 degrees.

Mix all ingredients together. Put in a glass or ceramic dish and bake for 30 minutes.

Serve with vegetables or whole-grain bread or crackers.

Nutritional analysis per serving

Serving size: About 1/2 cup

Calories123

Total fat3 g

Saturated fat1.5 g

Trans fat0 g

Monounsaturated fat1 g

Cholesterol6 mg

Sodium114 mg

Total carbohydrate16 g

Dietary fiber7.5 g

Added sugars0 g

Protein8 g